Keto Diet Guide For Beginners. 2019

Keto Diet
Meal,breakfast,lunch,dinner and
dessert

By

J.S. JOZEF

Volume 1

Copyright © 2019

Table of Contents

INTRODUCTION 7

CHAPTER ONE 8

What is a Ketogenic Diet? 8

What "keto" means 13

Possible therapeutic uses of the ketogenic diet........................ 16

History of Ketogenic Diet 20

CHAPTER TWO 22

The 7-Day Keto Meal Plan 22

CHAPTER THREE.. 42

Keto food preparation.. 42

Simple Steps for Easy Keto Meal Prep 52

Meal Prep Money Saving Tips.................................... 61

CHAPTER FOUR: 69

Keto breakfast recipes 69

CHAPTER FIVE 83

Keto Lunch Recipes 83

CHAPTER SIX 91

Keto dinner recipes 91

CHAPTER SEVEN.. 108

Keto Dessert Recipes 108

CHAPTER EIGHT 125

Frequently Asked Questions 125

CONCLUSION 131

Introduction

The world we live in is one where we have access to junk and unhealthy foods without stress, while healthy foods are cloaked to look very distasteful. Gone are those days when you had to sacrifice good taste, all in the name of eating healthily.

Have you heard so much about ketogenic lifestyle to the extent that you are wondering if it is worth the hype? Journey with us, and we will show you why you need to join those that are benefitting from this healthy diet.

Chapter one

What is a Ketogenic Diet?

For a lot of us that love to eat healthily, and lose weight, we must have heard of Ketogenic lifestyle. Day in, day out, you may wonder what ketogenic lifestyle is all about. You are in luck, as we will analyze every aspect.

One can say that the keto diet is one that integrates adequate protein and high fat, with very little carbs, and we won't be wrong.

The emphasis on the ketogenic diet is to reduce or strip your food of carbs while adding a high amount of fats to it.

When the ketogenic diet began, its creators weren't interested in using it to lose weight initially but had something in mind for it.

Ketogenic lifestyle was created to help treat epilepsy in kids. When a person consumes more and more of fats, the carbs that were once occupying a large part of the body mass is burnt. It gets to the stage, where the body no longer has carbs or glucose to burn. Hence it opts for the stored fat. The body focuses on the fat, burning it to act as a source of energy.

Usually, when a person is not subscribing to the ketogenic lifestyle, the person may tend to consume foods that are high in carbs. These carbs are turned to glucose. The glucose is moved around the body system, and it is used as fuel. The brain needs fuel to function.

When a person embraces a ketogenic lifestyle, his or her diet has little or no carbs. The body is forced to use the stored up fat as fuel.

The liver is forced to turn the fats, at this moment, to ketones and fatty acids. The ketones act as an energy source or fuel for the brain.

These ketones are transported to the brain, and they take the place of glucose. This means that the brain can depend on ketones, the same way it depends on glucose as a fuel source.

Once the ketone level in the body is high, the body is said to be in a state of ketosis. At this state, you will notice that a person is reducing in weight. For those kids suffering from epilepsy, when they are in a state of ketosis, there is a reduced level of seizures.

Research has shown that about half of those living with epilepsy that used this diet form had the rate of their seizures reduced by about half. The results didn't even change when they quit the diet. The Atkins diet offered them similar effect too. Know a child or young person that has epilepsy? The ketogenic diet can help.

For those that were suffering from pediatric epilepsy, the normal diet that was prescribed to them had the right amount of protein to help the child grow, while still given the right amount of calories to be at the right height and weight for their age.

The first type of therapeutic keto meal was designed to treat epilepsy in the early 1920s. It was used a lot to treat the ailment, but its usage reduced when drugs like anticonvulsant medications were made.

Keto diet is usually created to have high fat and low carbs. What is done is that there is an exclusion of foods that are high in carbs like starchy veggies, fruits, pasta, bread, sugar, as well as butter.

What "keto" means

The word, 'keto' in the keto diet means that the body will be forced to make use of ketones, which are tiny fuel molecules. This acts as another fuel for the human body, and takes the place of glucose when it is not in the right amount.

These energy molecules called, 'ketones' are made only when you eat little carbs. This means that if you consume a high amount if carbs, ketones can't be produced.

While the fat in the food acts as the energy source, the excess protein is turned into blood sugar.

The liver is the organ that is used in producing ketones from fat. Those tiny molecules produced are then transported around the body, including the brain.

The brain is one organ that is always hungry. Hence it needs a lot of energy daily. It is unable to run on fats but is capable of working well on glucose or ketones.

Once your body realizes that you are on a ketogenic diet, it has no other choice but to opt for fat, as it is a source of fuel. Immediately the insulin level plunges because the consumption of carbs has reduced, burning of fat increases.

At this stage, it is a lot easier if your fat stores are accessed, and burnt off quite easily.

This is awesome if you have decided to shed weight, as it can help you lose the excess weight. It is also great if you want to curtail your hunger, and still, have the necessary supply of energy.

A lot of persons who subscribe to the ketogenic lifestyle can testify that they are always focused and alert.

Immediately the body has started churning out ketones; it belongs to a stage christened, 'ketosis.' A lot of persons get into this stage quickly by fasting, but it's unable to fast forever. Fasting comes with a lot of issues that may affect your health.

This is where the ketogenic diet comes into play. You can continue the ketogenic lifestyle for a long while, enter the state of ketosis, and stay there. The ketogenic diet will give you what you wish- losing weight.

Possible therapeutic uses of the ketogenic diet
The ketogenic diet has been linked to the treatment of quite several neurological disorders like Parkinson's disease, Alzheimer's disease, brain cancer, pain, autism, amyotrophic lateral sclerosis, and even sleep disorders.

Epilepsy

Like earlier said, epilepsy is ranked as one of the commonest neurological disorders, following the ailment, stroke. It is said to be affecting millions of persons all over the world. One obvious symptom of epilepsy is unprovoked and regular seizures.

Seizures usually happen when a person has seizures, and this could affect the functioning of the brain. When seizures occur, the senses, muscles, or even consciousness may be affected. In the worst cases, three of them are affected.

Sometimes, the seizure can be restricted to a part of the brain, and in this case, it is called focal. Sometimes, it may spread around the entire brain, and in this case, it is generalized. Once a person has a generalized seizure, he or she may lose consciousness.

Causes of Epilepsy

The neurological condition can happen because of some reasons.

A lot of them started in one's childhood.

When one says that the case of epilepsy is refractory, it means that it has refused to be treated. This is a case when you have tried out about three or so anticonvulsant drugs, and they have all seemed to fail.

Statistics show that over sixty percent of the patients are known to get the control that they wish over their epilepsy using the first drug prescribed to them. Thirty percent of those with epilepsy do not get the necessary control using drugs.

When they realize that the drugs have failed, other options can be used. Some opt for the ketogenic diet, vagus nerve stimulation, as well as epilepsy surgery.

History of Ketogenic Diet

Ketogenic Diet came into limelight as a means of treating epilepsy. A lot of persons in the past made use of fasting to treat epilepsy, and it came with a lot of negative effects. When these were realized, a new method- a ketogenic lifestyle was created. It was meant to recreate the same success that fasting had created as a form of treating epilepsy.

It was very popular when it was created down to the 1930s, but its popularity waned when new anticonvulsant medications were created.

A lot of those that have epilepsy are capable of controlling their seizures by the use of medications.

For those that haven't been able to get the needed control, other methods are used.

Chapter Two

The 7-Day Keto Meal Plan

It has been noted that the ketogenic diet may be used by a lot of persons today to shed weight, it still has more uses. For those that want to embrace the ketogenic lifestyle, they may face challenges of how to create their first seven days meal plan. They are not to be planned, as being a first-timer in a tradition can do that.

Like earlier said, the ketogenic diet must have high fat, low carbs, and moderate protein. If it doesn't have any of the following, then it is not a ketogenic diet. If for any reason, you consume a food that is high in carbs, you may no longer be in the state of ketosis.

Let's say that the food you consume daily is 1,600 calories; you should eat about 100 grams of protein. It shouldn't be more than that, but it can be less.

You should consume about twenty-five grams of carbs. The number of carbs you consume shouldn't be more than that, but it can be less, while the fat you consume should be about 125 grams.

You can decide to mix any meal that you see on different days. They mustn't religiously follow.

All in all, it is expected that the daily macros be adjusted to meet your body needs.

You are expected to eat one serving for the recipes penned down, except when you are told otherwise.

DAY 1 DIETS

For Breakfast, eat

Keto Brunch Spread. The fat should be about 38g. Protein should be about 17g. Carbs should be about 3g, while calories should be about 426.

For lunch, eat Crispy Skin Salmon with Pesto Cauliflower Rice.

Fat should be about 51g. Protein should be about 24g. Carbs about 10g. Calories about 647.

For dinner, eat Superfood Meatballs and Keto Creamed Spinach.

The fats should be about 36g. Protein about 36g, and carbs about 7g. The calories should be about 485.

The total amount of macros that should be contained for the day are:

For fat, it should be 125g.

For protein, it should be 87g.

For carbs, it should be 20g.

The total amount of calories should be 1558.

DAY 2 MEALS

For breakfast, you should eat Chocolate Pancakes with Blueberry Butter.

The fats should be about 50g.

The protein should be about 27g.

Carbs should be about 11.5g

The calories should be about 611.

For lunch, eat Turkey Sausage Frittata and four slices bacon.

They should be fried in a tablespoon of butter, and you can use a cup of coffee while eating them.

The fats should be about 50g.

The protein should be about 25g.

The carbs should be about 5.5g, while total calories are 572.

For dinner, try out Lemon Herb Low Carb Keto Meatloaf.

The fats should be about 29g.

The protein should be about 33g.

The fats should be about 2g, while calories are about 344.

For the entire day, you should have total macros of:

Fats should be 129g

Protein should be 85g

Carbs should be 19g

Calories should be 1,527.

DAY 3 MEALS

For Breakfast, you should consider eating Bacon, Egg & Cheese Breakfast Casserole.

The fat in it should be 38g.

The protein in it should be 43g.

The carbs in it should be 4g, while the number of calories in it should be 437.

For Lunch, you can try out White Turkey Chili. It should be cooked with a tablespoon of olive oil, and two cups of mixed leafy greens.

The number of fats should be 44.5g.

Protein should be 28.8g.

Fats should be 5.5g, while calories are 568.

For dinner, try out Portobello Bun Cheeseburger with Celeriac. Ensure that everything there has been oven fried, and spice it with Homemade Keto Mayo.

The amount of fat there should be 40g.

Protein should be 31g, while carbs should be 13g. The calories are 539.

The entire macros for the day's consumption should be:

122.5 grams for fat consumption,

102.8 grams for protein consumption, 20.5 grams for carbs consumption, and 1,544 total calories consumed.

DAY 4 MEALS

For breakfast, you can decide to go for Keto Power Breakfast Bowl.

The number of fats should be 27g.

Protein should be 10.5g.

Carbs should be 7g, and calories should be 305.

For lunch, you can try out the Crispy Cheesy Chicken Salad.

For fat, it should contain 36.5g.

For protein should be 55g.

For carbs, it should be 8g.

As for calories, the total should be 575.

For dinner, you should try out Grilled ribeye steak- Four ounces, Mixed leafy greens- Two cups, Grass fed butter- Two tablespoons, and Avocado oil- A tablespoon.

For fat, it should have 62g.

For protein, it should be 20g.

For carbs, it should be a gram, and as for calories, the total should be about 636.

For Dessert, try out MCT Fat Bomb.

The fats should be 8g.

Protein should be 1g.

Carbs should be 2g.

Total calories should be 81.

For the entire day, the macros should be 133.5 grams for fat. As for protein and the total calories, they should be 86.5g and 1597 respectively.

DAY 5 MEALS

For breakfast, try out Avocado Breakfast Bowl.

The fat should be about 40g.

Protein should be about 25g.

Carbs should be about 3g.

The total calories should be about 500.

For lunch, try out the Roasted Chicken Stacks.

The fat should be 25g.

The protein should be 34g.

The carbs should be 5.5g.

Calories should be 369.

For dinner, try out the Cheesy Broccoli Meatza

For fat, it should be 24g.

For protein, it should be 32g.

For carbs, it should be 7g.

For calories, it should be 375.

For dessert, try out Two Macadamia Nut Fat Bombs.

Fats should be 34g.

Protein should be 2g.

Carbs should be 4g, while calories are 200.

For the entire day, the macros should be 123 grams for fat.

For protein, it should be 93 grams.

For carbs, it should be 19.5 grams, and calories are 1,444.

DAY 6 MEALS

For breakfast, try out Acai Almond Butter Smoothie.

For fat, it should be 40g.

For protein, it should be 15g.

For carb, it should be 6g, and calories should be 345.

For lunch, try out Keto Beef Bulgogi.

For fat, it should be 18g.

For protein, it should be 25g.

For carbs, it should be 3g, while the total amount of calories are 242.

For a snack, try out one ounce of almonds, and one hard-boiled egg.

For fat, it should be 19g.

For protein, it should be 12g.

For carbs, it should be 3g. Calories are 241.

For dinner, try out Creamy Mushroom Chicken.

For fat, it should be 27g.

For protein, it should be 24g.

For carbs, it should 3g.

Total calories are 241.

For Dessert, try out the Keto Chocolate Mousse.

For fats, it should be 14g.

For protein, it should be 17.5g.

For carbs, it should be 6g.

The total calories are 248.

For the entire, the macros are meant to be 98 grams for fat,

93.5 grams for protein,

21 grams for carbs.

The total calories should be 1,410.

DAY 7 MEALS

For Breakfast, try out Keto Bulletproof Coffee.

The fat should be 31g.

The protein should be 1g.

The carb should be 0.5g, while total calories are 280.

For Lunch, try out Low Carb Crispy Keto "Fried" Chicken, then top it with a cup of steamed broccoli.

For fat, it is 37g.

For protein, it should be 33.5g.

For carbs, it should be 6.5g.

For calories, it should be 494.

For dinner, try out Low Carb Keto Lasagna.

For fats, it should be 21g.

For protein, it should be 32g.

For carbs, it should be 12g.

For the total calories, it should be 364.

For dessert, try out Collagen Mug Cake.

For fats, it should be 43.5g.

For protein, it should be 27g.

For carbs, it should be 4g.

Total calories should be 535.

The macros for the entire day are:

Fats should be 122.5g.

Protein should be 93.5g.

Carbs should be 23g.

The total calories are 1,673.

There is one thing that should be noted, you will rarely meet your daily macro goal, but you shouldn't be scared. What you should do as a rule is to ensure that your protein and carbs goals are met to an extent.

You can easily look at the numbers if you wish.

Since you now know how a ketogenic diet week should look like, planning the next week should be a lot easier.

Chapter three

Keto food preparation

Research-Backed Reasons to Meal Prep on Keto

A lot of persons have the wrong thought that only motivation can get them to lose weight, and when they realize that it is a fallacy, you see them adding more weight than when they decided to shed the weight.

Don't think it is only you that have gone through such. For years, I have heard people complain that they thought motivation could get them through. The basic truth remains that motivation isn't everything.

You can't be motivated every blessed minute in the day, and that's the basic truth.

If you want to succeed on this journey, there has to be some plan. You don't have to rely on motivation to get the job done solely. A study that was done by the British Journal of Health Psychology stated that about ninety percent of those that participated in an exercise that was scheduled was known to work weekly, even if it was just once while those that didn't have any exercise scheduled had problems exercising, even if it was once a week.

If after this, you still need reasons you need to get up and start the meal prep immediately, below are awesome reasons:

#1: MEAL PREP CONQUERS DECISION FATIGUE

Do you that decision fatigue is a real thing? How? You may ask. Have you ever wondered why the likes of Mark Zuckerberg, Obama, and even Steve Jobs, while alive, wear the same clothes daily? The stress that comes with picking out cloth is exhausting. Hence they just buy similar clothes. This stops them from having to decide on what they should have on.

Humans are known to have restricted willpower, and if they are made to make decisions regularly, they get bored of it. The next decision they make becomes a chore, and before you know it they start asking if they even made the right decision. What would have happened if they had opted for the alternative?

Researchers decided to see what made prisoners become paroled, and it was noticed that there was a trend. After looking at more than a thousand decisions, it was noticed that prisoners were released parole based on a trend. Based on the report published by the New York Times, those prisoners that came before the judge in the morning were able to receive paroles a lot. About 70% was given parole. While those prisoners that came later on in the day had to battle with about ten percent or even less, this means that paroles were given to prisoners, not because of their crimes, but when they arrived.

When we look at it, we can see that the number of decisions that the judge had made earlier on in the day had forced him to see other decisions that he was to make as unappealing. This is basic psychology.

Have you ever gone to an office in the afternoon for something, and you saw them all angry, and tired of you immediately you entered there. Have you also gone to that office another day in the morning, and realized that they were happy to meet you?

Why is this so? No one likes to make decisions after making a string of decisions.

The same way the judge's willpower was reduced when he continuously made decisions is the same way you get tired of making decisions after a while.

The reason some persons quit keto is not that it's not effective, but the fact that they have to make choices when it comes to their food becomes tiring.

How can they save themselves the stress? The answer is very simple. You can create a meal plan, and you are good to go.

Your meal plan reduces the number of choices that need to be made. This makes your willpower to remain intact. If you want to adopt a ketogenic lifestyle, you need a meal plan.

2. Meal Prep Allows You Save Both Money and Time

Do you know that a typical person spends a lot of time and money making decisions? Let's say you refused to make a meal plan; you won't know what you want to eat. Hence you may end up spending a lot more money and time than necessary. Smart persons try to make a meal plan for weeks at a stretch, as it allows them to budget. If you know that you will be eating this and this, you can easily buy them in bulk and store. For those foods that can be cooked and stored in the refrigerator. You can always bring them out and microwave when you want to eat.

This allows you to save time that would have been wasted in shopping daily, cooking every time or looking for what meal to eat.

Planning your meal stops you from wasting food. This could help you save your money, but it can do much more.

For those that believe in saving the environment, food wastage is something that we should try and avoid.

When you plan, you save yourself this stress.

Planning your meals allows you to know what you intend to buy, and make you stick to those things that are important. It allows you to know how much you should spend for your groceries weekly.

3. Preparing for meals help you to reach the state of ketosis.

One thing that a lot of persons face is calculating their macros. It can be annoying to calculate them. Meal prep can help.

When you have a meal plan, it is quite easy for you to know what your macro goals are, and stick to them. You don't just make decisions out of nowhere that could affect your macro goals.

Simple Steps for Easy Keto Meal Prep

Everyone doesn't have to follow the same path while making their meal preps. This is to act as a guideline when deciding what to eat.

Start by deciding what you intend to eat.

You should start on the first day of the week. Write the day down, and think of what you should eat then. Write them down for breakfast down to dinner. Do it for the next six days.

Make up your mind on what you will eat every day for breakfast, lunch, and dinner. This should also include the desserts or snacks you may wish to consume.

You can put it in a calendar if you wish. On the other hand, you can have it broken down to every day that week.

Find out the calories of the foods you have chosen, and their composition. Remember that the fat content should be the highest, followed by protein and carbs.

Write out how many persons will munch on the food, and if you intend to have leftovers that can be consumed the day after, or if a new food will be consumed daily.

Ensure that the meal is kept simple by you eating the same food more than once in a week. This will allow you to save on the time that will be spent cooking, and you can dine on the leftovers. If you don't have the time or money to make mee foods every time, this can save you the stress. If, on the other hand, you have the time and money, you can make new delicacy every time without stress.

It is important that you pen down the recipes for the food that you will want to prepare. Don't forget to pin down the ingredients that will be used to prepare it. This will allow you to know what you need to prepare the food. You can easily source for the ingredients in bulk at the store and save yourself the stress.

Some persons don't mind doing everything in a day, and there are others that like to divide up the work.

A tip that can be used to your advantage is to choose those recipes that are easy to make and come bearing a few ingredients. You can opt for those recipes that have similar ingredients. Hence you can use them to make different foods.

You can decide to opt for recipes that use the same veggies or meats.

This allows the shopping list to be a lot shorter, and food can be cooked quickly.

In the end, you will be left with a shorter shopping list.

Create The List, Then Shop

Now that you have chosen the recipes you want and their ingredients, you can have your shopping list compiled. Have them broken down into groups, and you can begin the list with those that you see immediately you enter into the grocery shop.

Don't forget to pen down the amount of ingredient you want, and ensure that your shopping revolves around the list. Opt for the whole foods, and try to avoid packaged foods.

A lot of packaged foods may claim to be keto friendly, but they are far from that.

One method that I have used for a long time to shop is to immediately walk towards the produce and butcher sections, without looking at the packaged foods. This prevents me from stocking up on packaged foods and ignoring fresh produce or meat.

Prepare Your Meals

A lot of persons feel that shopping is the difficult part of the process, while some others, feel that it is the stage of preparing the meals. For those that opt for the former, it is not surprising because a lot of persons hate the thoughts of leaving their home and heading to the store. The thought of pushing the trolley annoys them. To some others, it may be the fact that there are a lot of options available, and before you know it, they have stocked their trolleys with unnecessary things.

For those that feel that cooking is the problem. We won't blame them. Maybe, they don't have a flair for cooking or cooking seems scary for them. Whichever way, cooking shouldn't be scary, especially when you have the recipe in front of you.

Cooking is one tricky process, but once you get used to it, it becomes so simple that you can cook while you sleepwalk.

Below are some tips that should be considered:

Get out the recipe, and read it. Before you bring out anything or start doing anything, try and understand every process. This prevents you from being stuck at a place or making mistakes.

Let's say that in the recipe, it states that you should slow cook the chicken. This should be something that you do first before you think of chipping the veggies or having the cauliflower rice made. This ensures that time isn't wasted.

Take out every ingredient that you will need before you start cooking. Go to the pantry and bring them out. If they are in the fridge, do the same.

If the recipe needs the veggies to be chopped, or the meats to be pre-cooked, you should consider doing that. This allows you to use them when you want easily.

Immediately you are done preparing the meal; it is advisable to store them in different containers. This will allow the foods to stay for a while.

You can have every container labeled with a sticky note to allow you to remember what it contains. You should also pen what day the food is meant for, as well as when it was made, and even the macros.

Meal Prep Money Saving Tips

A lot of persons feel that eating healthily or subscribing to the ketogenic lifestyle. What of if we told you that this is a pure fallacy?

Keto lifestyle is a very affordable one if you know what to do, or what to seek for. If you want to save money, while you eat healthily, then these tips will help.

Opt for those recipes that have seasonal produce. The trick of shopping is buying mostly those things that are in season. Why is this so? When something is in season, it tends to be a lot cheaper, and available. During the season for a food item, you can purchase a large amount of it for little or nothing, but when out of season, the opposite is the case.

You will likely see a lot of them on sale. Go to the grocery store and purchase them. Ensure that you have where to store them to prevent them from going stale.

Head To The Farmer's Market. This is one place that you should frequent. Many grocery stores get their produce from farmers, and when you decide to cut the middlemen out, you can get fresh foods without paying a lot. You may think that there's no farmer's market near you, but I doubt that. All you need to do is ask, and you will find. When you get there, be friendly with those in the market, and you will get great deals on fresh foods, especially dairy products.

Stay off packaged foods

The truth remains that one can't stay off packaged food, but you can reduce the amount that you consume. Apart from the fact that packaged foods are far from healthy, they aren't cheap. You may say that they have been cleaned and bagged. Hence the are easier to use, but have you considered the hole that it is digging in your pocket.

They may seem convenient, but they aren't so affordable. You can get fresh food, and save yourself some money. Usually, when you compare how much you spend on processed foods and fresh ones, you will realize that the disparity is much.

Search around for coupons or discounts

Stores are known to churn out special offers, but you may not know of them. Some persons only find out when they search or head to the store.

You can visit the store's website to seek for those offers. To get a regular stream of such information, save yourself the trouble, and sign up for their email newsletters. It may seem like an inconvenience, but you won't know when you will get those deals.

Purchase in the large amount

This is a smart trick that buyers have used for a long time. When items are being purchased in bulk, discounts are given to the buyer. You can head to the farmer's market or grocery store and purchase the ingredients in bulk. Before you do this, it is important that you have where to store them. Don't go and buy those items that will end up spoiling because you don't have storage space.

Have your items grown

If you fall under those with green thumbs, you will enjoy growing your food. It will help you save money that would have been expended in a store. Forget about the money saved, do you know that it is healthier to consume home grown foods than the one bought in the store? A lot of store foods are genetically modified and have been stripped of part of their nutrients. Some are toxic to the body because of the chemicals that have been added to grow them.

If you have a yard, you should think of growing herbs and veggies there. You don't have to have a big yard before you can do it. There are currently a lot of space managing tips online that help those with tiny space grow their foods.

You can also make your food. Yes, you read that right. Instead of heading to the store to get the processed varieties, you can make things like

- Mayo,

- Bone broth,

- Ketchup,

- Salad dressings and sauces,

- Bacon,

- Mustard,

- Sauerkraut,

- Pesto,

- Ghee,

- Coconut flour,

- Almond milk and so on.

There are tips on how to make them online.

Chapter Four:

Keto breakfast recipes

We have discussed some life-saving tips that you can use to lead a healthy lifestyle without breaking the bank. Now, we will look at those healthy ketogenic breakfast recipes that you should consider.

A lot of persons believe that keto recipes have to stale to the tongue. Far from it, keto wants you to lead a healthy lifestyle, and it also wants you to eat delicious foods. You may have shied away from other healthy lifestyles because of how averse they were to the taste bud, but this is different.

Keto cereal

You can treat your taste buds to the good things of life, and treat your body to a healthy diet. All you have to do is try out the keto cereal, and you will be impressed.

What You Need

- Chopped Almonds- One c.

- Sesame seeds- Quarter c.

- Walnuts- One c.

- Unsweetened coconut flakes- One c.

- Chia seeds- Two tablespoons

- Flax seeds- Two tablespoons

- Ground clove- One and a half teaspoon

- Cinnamon- One and a half teaspoon

- Egg white- One

- Kosher salt- Half teaspoon

- Coconut oil- Quarter c

- Cooking spray

Directions

Start by having the oven preheated to 250. Get out your baking sheet, and line it with cooking spray.

Take out a big bowl, and toss in your coconut flakes, almonds, flax seeds, sesame seeds, walnuts, as well as chia seeds.

Whisk in your vanilla, cinnamon, salt, as well as cloves.

Whisk the egg white till it becomes foamy, then add it to the granola. Whisk in the coconut oil, and don't stop until they are coated well.

Put the mixture on the baking sheet, and ensure that it is well layered.

Allow it bake for about twenty-five minutes. Ensure that it is golden before you bring it out. Allow it cool well before you serve.

Best-Ever Cabbage Hash Browns

What You Need

- Kosher salt- Half teaspoon

- Eggs- Two

- Galic powder- Half teaspoon

- Pepper- to taste

- Vegetable oil- One tablespoon

- Yellow onion- Quarter

- Shredded cabbage- Two c.

Directions

Get out a big bowl and stir your garlic powder, eggs, and salt. Toss in the black pepper, before you add the onion and cabbage. Ensure you mix well, and don't stop.

Take out a big skillet, and put it on a stove with medium heat. Add your oil, and allow it heat for a while.

Have the mixture divided into four patties in that pan that you have decided to use? Make use of your spatula and have them flattened. Allow them to cook till they become tender and golden for over three minutes. You should then turn to the other side.

Keto pancakes

What You Need

- Almond flour- Half c
- Eggs- Four
- Cream cheese- Four ounces
- Lemon zest- One teaspoon.
- Butter

Directions

Take out a medium bowl, and stir in the eggs, cream cheese, lemon zest, and almond flour. Continue to stir till they become smooth.

Take out your nonstick skillet and place it on a stove with medium heat. Have a tbsp of butter melted on it, then add three tablespoons of the batter. Allow them to cook for about two minutes or till you notice that they have taken the golden hue.

Toss them to the other side, and allow them to cook for about two minutes again.

Put them in a plate, then continuously cook the rest of the batter.

You can top them with butter.

Keto smoothie

What You Need

- Strawberries- Two c.

- Raspberries- Two c

- Blackberries- Two c

- Baby spinach- One c

- Coconut milk- Two c

- Orange juice

- Unsweetened shaved coconut. This is to garnish. Hence it is optional.

Directions

Take out a blender and add all these ingredients. Leave the coconut out of the mixture. Blend them till you notice that they are smooth.

Take out your cups and fill. You can garnish them with coconut and raspberries.

Keto breakfast cup

What You Need

- Ground pork- Two lb

- Chopped thyme- One tablespoon

- Garlic- Two cloves

- Paprika- Half teaspoon

- Cumin- Half teaspoon

- Salt- One teaspoon

- Fresh spinach- Chopped.

- Two and a half c

- Black pepper- to taste

- Shredded cheddar- One c

- Eggs- Twelve

- Chopped chives- A tablespoon

Directions

Start by preheating the oven until it reaches a temperature of 200. Take out a big bowl, and add your cumin, paprika, garlic, thyme, ground pork, as well as salt. Toss in the pepper.

Take out a bit of the pork and place them on every muffin tin. Have every side pressed up to form a cup. Have the cheese and spinach divided up well among the cups?

Get an egg, and crack it on every cup. Add pepper and salt to taste. Do the same for the remaining eggs.

Leave them in the oven, and allow them to bake well. This should take over twenty-five minutes. Add your chives, then serve.

Keto blueberry muffin

What You Need

- Almond flour- Two and a half c.

- Sugar- One-third c. Keto friendly

- Baking powder- One and a half teaspoons

- Salt- Half teaspoon

- Baking soda- Half teaspoon

- Melted butter- One this c.

- Almond milk- One third c

- Eggs- Three

- Vanilla extract- A teaspoon

- Blueberries- One teaspoon

- Lemon zest- Half

- Blueberries- Two-third c.

Directions

Have your oven preheated to 150. Take out your muffin pan, and line it with cupcake liners.

Take out a big bowl, and toss in your Swerve, almond flour, salt, baking soda, baking powder.

Toss in your eggs, almond milk, butter, and vanilla. Don't stop until they are well mixed

Take out the lemon zest and blueberries and fold till well distributed.

Take out similar amounts of the batter in the cupcake liner, and put in the oven. Allow it bake for about twenty-three minutes. To be sure that they are ready, you can use a toothpick and insert it in the muffin. If it comes out clean, then it is ready.

Allow them to cool well before you serve.

Chapter Five

Keto Lunch Recipes

Loaded cauliflower bake

What You Need

- Cauliflower head- One. Cut to form florets
- Butter- Two tablespoons
- Heavy cream- One cup
- Cream cheese- Two ounces
- Sharp cheddar- One and quarter cup
- Pepper and salt
- Bacon- Six slices
- Green onions- Quarter cup

Directions

Start by preheating the oven until it reaches a high temperature of 150.

Take out a big pot and boil water. When it is boiling, put the cauliflower florets there for two minutes. After then, have the cauliflower drained.

Take out a medium pot, and melt the cream cheese, heavy cream, and butter. Stir in the pepper salt and cheddar cheese. Don't stop till they are well combined.

Take out your baking dish, and toss in the cheese sauce, cauliflower florets, then add every crumbled bacon and green onions, but save one tablespoon of each somewhere else. Stir the mixture together.

Add the extra crumbled bacon, cheddar cheese and green onions to them.

Allow them to bake till the cheese has become golden and bubbly. The cauliflower must be soft before you bring it out. This should take about thirty minutes.

Turkey Chili

What You Need

- Organic ground turkey- One lb

- Cauliflower- Two cups

- Coconut oil- Two tablespoons

- Vidalia onion- Half

- Garlic- Two cloves

- Coconut milk- Two cups

- Mustard- A tablespoon

- Salt- One teaspoon

Directions

Start by heating the coconut oil in a big pot.

While it heats, cut the garlic and onion, then put them in the hot oil.

Continue to stir them for about two minutes before you put the ground turkey.

Have the mixture broken up using the spatula. Dong stop stirring till you see that it is crumbled.

Put the seasoning mix, as well as the riced cauliflower. Don't forget to stir well.

When you notice that the meat is now browned, put the coconut milk, and allow it to simmer for about eight minutes. Don't forget to stir.

Once it gets to this point, you can then serve. Add the shredded cheese to give it the thick sauce feel.

BBQ pulled beef Sando

Who said you have to eat bland foods all in the name of leading a ketogenic lifestyle? No one. Bask in the good things of life, and tasty foods with the BBQ pulled beef Sando.

What You Need

- Boneless Chuck Roast- Three lbs
- Pink Himalayan Salt- Two teaspoons
- Garlic powder- Two teaspoons
- Black pepper- One teaspoon
- Onion powder- One teaspoon
- Smoked paprika- One tablespoon
- Tomato paste- Two tablespoons
- Apple cider vinegar- Quarter cup
- Coconut aminos- Two tablespoons

- Bone broth- Half cup

- Butter- Quarter cup

Directions

Have the fat trimmed off the beef, before you cut them up into two big pieces.

Take out a small bowl, then toss in the ingredients like black pepper, onion, salt, paprika, and garlic. Leave the beef to cook in a slow cooker.

Take out another bowl, and have the butter melted. Don't forget to add the vinegar, tomato paste, as well as coconut aminos. Pour the mixture on the beef.

Allow it to cook for about ten hours, but it should be on low. When it is ready, take out the beef, and leave the slow cooker at a high temperature. This will allow it thicken. You can then have the beef shredded before you add it to the slow cooker. Put the sauce, and voilà, you are good to go.

You can then serve.

Chapter Six

Keto dinner recipes

Want to dine with your family healthily, yet satisfy your taste buds? Try out the following keto dinner recipes. They are affordable and easy to make.

Bell pepper eggs

What You Need

- Bell pepper- One

- Eggs- Six

- Kosher salt

- Black peppers

- Chopped chives- Two tablespoons

- Chopped parsley- Two tablespoons

Directions

Take out a skillet, and place it on a stove with medium heat. Ensure that you grease it well with cooking spray.

Take out the bell pepper ring and put in the skillet. Allow it sauté for about two minutes. Ensure that the ring is flipped before you crack the egg there in the middle.

Put your pepper and salt to season it, then allow it to cook for about three minutes, till you notice that egg has been cooked.

Do the same thing with the remaining eggs, and don't forget to have them garnished with parsley and chives.

Bunless bacon, egg, and cheese

What You Need

- Eggs- Twp
- Water- Two tablespoons
- Avocado- Half
- Cooked bacon- Two slices
- Cheddar cheese- Quarter C.

Directions

Take out a medium pan, and put two mason jar lids there. Ensure that you have removed the centers.

Using cooking spray, spray the pan, and put it on a stove with medium heat.

Bring the eggs, and have them cracked in the middle of the lids. Try and whisk it lightly using a fork to remove the yolk.

Around the lids, pour water and have the pan covered. Allow them to cook for a while till you notice that the whites have been cooked.

Take out the lid, and add the cheddar on the eggs. Allow them to cook until they become a bit melty. This can take about a minute.

Have the egg bun inverted on a plate without the cheese. Have it topped with cooked Bacon, as well as mashed avocado.

Top it using the cheesy egg bun, while the cheese faces side-down. You can munch on them with a fork and knife.

Cloud eggs

What You Need

- Eggs- Eight

- Parmesan- One c

- Deli ham- Half Lb

- Black pepper

- Kosher salt

- Chopped chives

Directions

Start by preheating the oven until it gets to 250.

Have the baking sheet greased with cooking spray.

Get the yolks and egg whites separated. Put the egg whites in a big bowl, and yolk in the small bowl. Use a hand mixer to whisk the egg whites for about three minutes or till you notice that stiff peaks have formed.

Add in the ham and Parmesan, then season with a bit of pepper and salt.

Take out about eight mounds of the egg whites into the baking sheet, and indent the centers to create nests. Allow them to bake for three minutes till you notice that they are golden.

Before you serve, garnish them with chives.

Cookie dough keto fat bomb

What You Need

- Butter- Eight tablespoons

- Keto friendly sweetener like Swerve- One-third c.

- Vanilla extract- Half teaspoon

- Kosher salt- Half teaspoon

- Almond flour- Two c

- Chocolate chips- Two third c

Directions

Take out a big bowl, and put the butter there. Beat it with a hand mixer till you notice that it is fluffy and light. Toss in the salt, vanilla, and sugar. Continue to beat till they combine well.

Gently whisk in the almond flour till you can't see any dry spot again. Add the chocolate chips.

Use a plastic wrap to cover the bowl, and leave it in the refrigerator for about twenty minutes to become quite firm.

Make use of a tiny cookie scoop to scoop the dough till it forms tiny balls. Leave it in the fridge, and it can stay for up to a week. If you want it to stay up to a month, leave in the freezer.

Bacon avocado bomb

What You Need

- Avocado- Two
- Bacon- Eight

- Cheddar- One third c

Directions

Start by heating the broiler. Take out your baking sheet, and have it lined with foil.

Have the avocado sliced into half, then take out the pits. Remove the skin from every avocado.

Ensures that the halves are filled with cheese, then put the other halves of the avocado. Have every avocado wrapped with bacon- four slices.

Put the avocado now wrapped in bacon in the baking sheet, and allow it broil till you notice that the bacon is now crispy. This should take about five minutes.

Gently, turn the avocado with tongs, and allow them to cook till crispy. This should take an extra five minutes.

Plain Cloud Bread

What You Need

- Three eggs
- Cream of tartar- Quarter teaspoon
- Kosher salt- A pinch
- Cream cheese- Two ounces

Directions

Start by preheating the oven to a high temperature of 200. Have your baking sheet lined with the parchment paper.

Take out two bowls, and separate the yolks from the egg whites. Put the salt and cream of tartar to the egg whites. Use a hand mixer to whisk well till you notice the stiff peaks. This should take about three minutes.

Toss in the cream cheese to egg yolks. Take out your hand mixer and whisk the cream cheese with the mix yolks till you notice that they are well combined. Gradually pour the egg yolk mixture to the egg whites.

Have the mixture divided into six mounds on the baking sheet. Ensure that they have been spaced about four inches away. Continue to bake for thirty minutes till you notice that they are golden.

Have each bread piece sprinkled with cheese. Leave it in the oven to bake for about two minutes, till the cheese melts.

Allow it cool before you serve.

Pizza Cloud Bread

What You Need

- Italian seasoning- One tablespoon
- Shredded mozzarella- Two tablespoons

- Parmesan- Two tablespoons

- Tomato paste- Two teaspoons

Directions

Break the egg, and put a tbsp of Italian seasoning, tomato paste, shredded mozzarella into the egg yolk mixture

Have the mixture divided into six mounds on the baking sheet. Ensure that they have been spaced about four inches away. Continue to bake for thirty minutes till you notice that they are golden.

Have each bread piece sprinkled with cheese. Leave it in the oven to bake for about two minutes, till the cheese melts.

Allow it cool before you serve.

Bagel Cloud Bread

What You Need

- Kosher salt- One-eight teaspoon

- Poppy seeds- One teaspoon

- Sesame seeds- One teaspoon

- Dried garlic- One teaspoon

- Dried onion- One teaspoon. Minced

Directions

Break the egg, and put it in a bowl. Add the poppy seeds, kosher salt, sesame seed, dried onion, and dried garlic to the mixture.

Have the mixture divided into six mounds on the baking sheet. Ensure that they have been spaced about four inches away. Continue to bake for thirty minutes till you notice that they are golden.

Have each bread piece sprinkled with cheese. Leave it in the oven to bake for about two minutes, till the cheese melts.

Allow it cool before you serve.

Ranch Cloud Bread

- Ranch seasoning powder- One and a half teaspoons
- Eggs

Directions

Break the egg in a big bowl, and add the ranch seasoning powder into the egg yolk mixture.

Have the mixture divided into six mounds on the baking sheet. Ensure that they have been spaced about four inches away. Continue to bake for thirty minutes till you notice that they are golden.

Have each bread piece sprinkled with cheese. Leave it in the oven to bake for about two minutes, till the cheese melts.

Allow it cool before you serve.

Chapter Seven

Keto Dessert Recipes

Keto diets also come in the form of desserts. This means that you can enjoy your dessert recipe without stress.

Keto avocado brownies

What You Need

- Eggs- Four

- Avocados- Two

- Butter- Half c. Melted

- Peanut butter- Six tablespoons- Six

- Baking soda- Two teaspoons

- Coconut sugar- Two- third c.

- Vanilla extract- Two teaspoons

- Cocoa powder- Two teaspoons

- Salt- Half teaspoon

Directions

Start by preheating the oven to a high temperature of 250. Get out your pan out, and have it lined with parchment paper. Take out your blender and toss in every ingredient, then blend till you notice that it is smooth.

Put the batter in the baking pan, and make use of a spatula to smoothen it.

Leave in the oven till you notice that the brownies are now soft, but they shouldn't be wet. This usually takes about twenty-five minutes. Before you serve, allow them to cool.

Chocolate mousse

What You Need

- Avocados- Two

- Heavy dream- Three-quarter c.

- Chocolate chips- Half c. Must be keto friendly.

- Honey- Quarter c

- Cocoa powder- Three tablespoons. Unsweetened.

- Honey- Quarter c.

- Kosher salt- Half teaspoon

Directions

Take out your blender and toss in every ingredient. Don't put the chocolate yet.

Blend them, toss in the chocolate, then blend again.

Pour it in your glasses, and allow it to sit in the refrigerator for a while before you serve.

Keto frosty

What You Need

- Whipping cream- One and a half c.

- Cocoa powder- Two tablespoons

- Sugar sweetener- Three tablespoons. Keto friendly

- Kosher salt- A pinch

- Vanilla extract- A teaspoon

Directions

Take out a big bowl, and toss in your salt, vanilla, sweetener, cocoa, and cream. Use a hand mixer and beat it till you notice stiff peaks forming. Take out your Ziploc bag, and pour the mixture in. Allow it freeze for thirty minutes.

Snip a part of the bag out, and put in the serving dishes.

Magic keto cookies

What You Need

- Coconut oil- Quarter c

- Butter- Four tablespoons. Softened

- Swerve sweetener- Two tablespoons

- Egg yolks- Four

- Coconut flakes- One c

- Dark chocolate chips- One c

- Coconut flakes- One c

- Chopped Walnuts- Three third c.

Directions

Start by preheating the oven until it reaches a high temperature of 250.

Take out a baking sheet, and have it lined with parchment paper.

Take out a big bowl, and whisk in egg yolks, sweetener, butter, and coconut oil. Add your walnuts, coconut and chocolate chips.

Put the batter into the baking sheet, and leave in the oven. Allow it to bake for about fifteen minutes or till it becomes golden.

Peanut butter cookies

What You Need

- Unsweetened Peanut- One and a half c

- Coconut flour- One c.

- Coconut sugar- Quarter c.

- Vanilla extract- One teaspoon

- Kosher salt- A pinch

- Chocolate chips- Two c.

- Coconut oil- A tablespoon

Directions

Take out a medium bowl, and toss in the salt, vanilla, coconut sugar, coconut flour, and peanut butter.

Take out your baking sheet and line with parchment paper. Make use of a tiny cookie scoop, and form the mixture to rounds before you press them down on the baking sheet. This will flatten them. Allow them to freeze for about one hour, or till you notice that it is firm.

Take out a medium bowl, and toss in the coconut oil and melted chocolate.

Making use of a fork, dip the rounded peanut butter in the chocolate till you notice that it has been properly coated. Take it back to the baking sheet.

Pour more peanut butter on them, and allow them to freeze till you notice that they are set. This usually takes ten minutes.

You can then serve cold. Allow them to stay in the freezer.

Chocolate mug cake

What You Need

- Butter- Two tablespoons

- Egg- One

- Cocoa powder- Two tablespoons

- Almond flour- Quarter c

- Chocolate chips- Two tablespoons. Keto friendly

- Baking powder- Half teaspoon

- Keto friendly sweetener- One teaspoon

- Kosher salt- A pinch

- Whipped cream- Quarter c

Directions

Take out a safe microwave mug and coat it with butter. Allow it to stay in a microwave for thirty seconds to melt. Put the other ingredients, and not the whipped cream. Continue to stir till you notice that they are fully mixed.

Allow it to cook for about a minute, till the cake is now set, but still having the fudgy feel.

Garnish with whipped cream.

You can then serve.

Keto ice cream

What You Need

- Coconut milk- Two. Fifteen ounces

- Heavy cream- Two c

- Sweetener- Keto friendly. Quarter c

- Vanilla extract- One teaspoon

- Kosher salt- A pinch.

Directions

Start by chilling the coconut oil in the refrigerator for about three hours. You can do it overnight.

Take out the coconut cream, and pour it in a big bowl. Leave the remaining liquid in the can.

Take out a hand mixer and beat till it is very creamy. Allow it rest.

Take out a big bowl, and use a mixer to beat the heavy cream till you notice that soft peaks have formed. You can then whisk in the vanilla and sweetener.

Whisk the whipped coconut to the whipped cream, then toss them in the loaf pan.

Allow them to freeze for close to five hours.

Sugar-free cheesecake

What You Need

- Almond flour- Half c

- Coconut flour- Half c

- Shredded coconut- Quarter c

- Melted butter- Half c

- Cream cheese- Three. Eight ounces

- Sour cream- Sixteen ounces

- Stevia- One tablespoon

- Pure vanilla extract- Two teaspoons

- Eggs- Three

- Strawberries- Sliced.

Directions

Start by preheating the oven to 200.

Start to make the crust:

Take out your spring form pan, and grease it, before covering the edges and bottoms with foil.

Take out a medium bowl, and toss in the butter, coconut and flours. Put the crust into the pan's bottom, and let it move to the sides of the pan.

Leave the pan in the refrigerator for a period. Use this time to have the filling made.

Have the filling made:

Take out a big bowl, and toss in the sour cream and cream cheese. Beat them, then whisk in the vanilla and stevia.

Toss in the eggs, and mix them. Ensure that the filling is spread well on the crust.

Leave the cheesecake in the pan, and put it in the middle rack of the oven.

Be careful as you pour boiling water in the pan till it reaches halfway.

Allow it bake for about one hour, till you notice that it jiggles lightly in the middle. Switch off the oven, but let the cake sit in the oven. Keep the door open a bit for one hour.

Take out the pan from its water bath, and remove the foil.

Leave it in the refrigerator for about five hours.

You can throw in some strawberries as garnish.

Chapter Eight

Frequently Asked Questions

Keto Adaptation- What Is It, And How Does It Feel Like?

What keto-adaption means is that your body has moved from using glucose as an energy source to using ketones.

It usually takes a few weeks after you start your keto diet before you notice this. This is if you flow it religiously. At first, you may see some symptoms that come with carbohydrate withdrawal, but all that change when you get used to it.

Keto flu: What is it? Is it avoidable?

The body normally needs glucose for its energy source. When the body realizes that you have cut carbs, it ma freak out, and this can be shown in keto flu. Some persons may not notice it, and others may. You may start to notice some flu symptoms, but it is for a very short while. Drink enough water, and you will be alright.

How long does it take to become keto-adapted or in a state of ketosis?

Research has shown that it takes a few weeks, and it can reach four weeks.

If you can cut out carbs, you can reach there quicker. If you want to speed the process, you can also exercise. Exercise will force the body to use its stored up fat.

What does ketosis mean?

When you are in the state of ketosis, your liver is creating a large number of ketones, which the body, especially the brain uses as an energy source or fuel. To work out well, you need to reduce your carbs drastically, while consuming a high amount of fats, and moderate protein.

How can I tell if I am in ketosis?

It is quite easy to tell, though you can use a breathalyzer to test it or carry out a urine or blood test to know for sure.

If you are in a state of ketosis, you will notice that your mouth is now metallic and fruity. This is what is known as keto breath. This shows that your body is running on ketones.

You will realize that you have become a lot more alert and sharp.

What may make me lose the state of ketosis, and how can I get back into it quickly?

It is hard to get into the state of ketosis, but a lot easier. The moment you eat a food that is high in carbs, your body will no longer be in a state of ketosis. The human body is wired to use glucose as an energy source. Immediately it sees carbs; it makes use of it. You can get back to ketosis by doing the same thing that got you there in the first place.

Do I need to incorporate carbohydrate re-feed days?

There are varying kinds of keto diets, and some offer you the necessary flexibility to add carb re-feed days.

These are great for those that are just starting keto diet, those that are active and need carbs for their workout, and those that had no choice but to eat carbs once in a while because of their social environment.

What is the difference between a low-carbohydrate diet and a ketogenic diet?

Don't confuse low carb foods and ketogenic diets. Consuming foods that contain close 150 grams of carbs daily can be said to be low carbs, but ketogenic needs something else.

To be in ketosis, you need to consume carbs of below 50g. Keto diet is moderate in protein and high in fat.

Conclusion

On your journey to eating healthily or shedding weight, one thing is sure; Ketogenic lifestyle can help. Gone are those days when you had to spend all your money drinking one pill or the other and pumping yourself with harmful substances all in the name of trying to lose weight. Ketogenic lifestyle can offer you this without you spending a lot of money. What else are you awaiting? Eat healthily and shed weight, without sacrificing good taste.